Ultimate Gluten-Free Diet Cookbook!

Gluten-Free

The Beginners Guide To Living The Gluten-Free Lifestyle With Easy Gluten-Free Recipes And Suggestions For Eating Healthy And Cheap!

Sarah Brooks

STOP!!! Before you read any further....Would you like to know the Secrets of Body Transformation?

If your answer is yes, then you are not alone. Thousands of people are looking for the secret to rapidly burn body fat, keep the weight off, become healthier, and truly transform their body and life for good.

If you have been searching for these answers without much luck, you are in the right place!

Not only will you gain incredible insight in this book, but because I want to make sure to give you as much value as possible, right now for a limited time you can get full **100% FREE access to a VIP bonus EBook** entitled **THE 7 KEYS TO BODY TRANSFORMATION!**

Just Go Here For Free Instant Access:

www.liveFitVIP.com

Legal Notice

Disclaimer Notice

Table Of Contents

Introduction

I want to thank you and congratulate you for purchasing the book, *"Gluten-Free: Ultimate Gluten-Free Diet Cookbook! The Beginners Guide To Living The Gluten-Free Lifestyle With Easy Gluten-Free Recipes And Suggestions For Eating Healthy And Cheap!"*

This "Gluten-Free" book contains proven steps and strategies on how to live a healthier life without the harmful effects of gluten. It also contains tips on how to live a gluten-free life without harming your budget.

In this book, you will find:

- Easy Gluten-Free recipes fit for beginners.
- Delicious and refreshing Gluten-free desserts and smoothies
- Gluten-free Paleo diet recipes and smoothies
- Gluten-free substitutes that are good for the body
- Gluten-free recipes that help balance blood sugar in the body.

A lot of people suffer from Celiac disease and gluten sensitivity. If you are one of them, you will benefit greatly from this book. The recipes contained in this cookbook can also benefit those suffering from diabetes. Or, if you are looking for a diet that will help you lose weight and simply make you healthier, this cookbook is just what you need.

So, start learning the benefits of a Gluten-free living and reap the benefits of having a healthier body all the time.

Thanks again for purchasing this book, I hope you enjoy it!

Chapter 1 - What Is Gluten: Benefits Of A Gluten-free Lifestyle

Gluten is a combination of two proteins, gliadin and glutenin, which acts as a glue for foods to maintain their shape and stick together. Gluten also makes the dough elastic and helps make it rise. Oftentimes, gluten is also responsible for the chewy texture of the final product.

Gluten is commonly found in wheat, barley, rye and products containing them. Due to the properties of gluten, it is also commonly used in many dermatological preparations, cosmetics and hair products. Globally, gluten is used as a source of protein from foods prepared using products containing it or as an additive to low-protein foods.

Going on a gluten-free diet has a lot of health benefits. When you go gluten-free, you are also eliminating various unhealthy foods such as fried foods and high sugar, high fat pastries and desserts. As a result, your cholesterol level is improved, your energy levels are increased and your digestive health is better.

Going gluten-free also means you will consume more fruits and vegetables since they are completely gluten-free and they are also non-starchy. This means you are getting rid of processed foods that are full of chemicals and are essentially bad for your health.

Even those who do not suffer from celiac disease or gluten intolerance have reported that they feel healthier and better after going on a gluten-free diet. This is mainly because they are eating healthier, non-processed foods that are very nutritious and low in fat and calories. This is why most health enthusiasts and dietitians recommend gluten-free diet for those who want to lose weight.

Chapter 2 - The Effects Of Gluten In Our Body

People diagnosed with celiac disease and gluten insensitivity are increasing. celiac disease is an autoimmune ailment that affects the digestive system. When celiac sufferers consume products with gluten, their immune system responds by destroying the villi (tiny, finger-like protrusions) found in the small intestines. This disease is detected through blood testing.

Early symptoms of this disease include bloating, gas, stomach pain, weight loss, and decrease in appetite, constant or intermittent diarrhea, floating stools that appear bloody or fatty and vomiting.

Gluten intolerance, on the other hand is not an autoimmune disease. When a person with gluten intolerance consumes any product containing gluten, it causes bloating, abdominal cramping, flatulence and diarrhea.

Gluten sensitivity is a less harmful form of gluten intolerance. Although the symptoms are the same with celiac disease, gluten sensitivity does not damage the intestinal lining.

If you experience any of the symptoms above after consuming products containing gluten, chances are, you may be gluten intolerant. You should consult your doctor right away for proper diagnosis. It is important that you stick on the same diet that you have before you visit the doctor to ensure an objective test result. Celiac disease is not easy to diagnose and if you switch in a different diet before you go for testing, the results may not be reliable.

Chapter 3 - Gluten-Free Diet For Beginners

If you are new to the gluten-free diet, you should know which products are allowed and which ones are not. Below is a list to help guide beginners like you in your journey to the gluten-free diet.

Products that are not allowed:

- Wheat – It includes Graham, Couscous, Bulgur, Durum, Einkorn, Kamut, Farro, Spelt, Matzo Meal and Semolina. Modified wheat starch, wheat starch, pregelatinized wheat protein

- Rye – This grain is commonly found in sandwich breads such as pumpernickel bread and bread with caraway seeds.

- Barley – This grain is also used for making malt flavoring. Malt vinegar is also made from fermented barley so it is not gluten-free.

- Triticale – This grain is a crossbreed of rye and wheat. It is used in brewing, distilling, bread and cereal manufacturing.

All derivatives of these grains also contain gluten so you have to watch out for them as well. Breads, pastries, pastas, breading and coating mix, energy bars, flour or cereal products, salad dressings, sauces and gravies, roux, marinades and many other products also contain gluten.

Products that are allowed:

- Corn – All forms of corn are allowed (cornmeal, grits, corn flour, etc.).

- Rice – Rice and all its forms are allowed (brown, white, enriched rice, basmati, etc.).

- Amaranth

- Buckwheat (Kasha)

- Montina

- Millet

- Quinoa

- Teff

- Sorghum

- Soy

Products such as butter, milk, real cheese, margarine, plain yoghurt and vegetable oils are all gluten-free. Fruits and vegetables, meat, eggs, seafood, beans, nuts and legumes are also gluten-free including the flours made from them.

However, note that gluten-free food products may also be contaminated with gluten through cross-contamination so you have to be careful. This happens during manufacturing wherein the gluten-free product gets in contact with products containing gluten.

Chapter 4 - Easy And Budget Friendly Gluten-free Recipes

Going gluten-free can also be budget friendly. Follow these deliciously simple Gluten-free recipes without hurting your budget.

Gluten-Free Stuffed Tomatoes

Ingredients:

8 large Tomatoes, cut on top, flesh removed (reserve for later use)

2 ½ cups Brown Rice, cooked

4 Shallots, finely chopped (pale part only)

75 grams Feta (reduced-fat), crumbled

¼ cup Currants

2 tablespoons fresh Mint, chopped

2 tablespoon fresh Parsley, chopped

½ teaspoon Cinnamon, ground

A bunch of Rocket, trimmed

1 tablespoon Balsamic Vinegar

Olive Oil spray

Salt to taste

Directions:

1. Preheat oven to 180° Celsius. Line your baking tray with non-stick baking paper.

2. Line the tomatoes in a paper towel, cut-side facing down. Strain the flesh into a bowl using a fine sieve. You will need about ½ cup of tomato juice.

3. Mix together cooked brown rice, feta, shallots, mint, currants, cinnamon, parsley and tomato juice in a large bowl. Season with salt and pepper.

4. Stuff the rice mixture into the tomato shells. Line each tomato shells on the baking tray. Spray lightly with olive oil. Bake for 10 minutes.

5. Cover with the cut tomato tops and bake for another 5 minutes. Do not overcook so the tomatoes won't lose their shape.

6. In another bowl, combine vinegar and rocket. Serve cooked stuffed tomatoes with salad on the side.

Fluffy Prosciutto Omelet

Ingredients:

240 grams Cherry Truss Tomatoes, washed and drained

1 teaspoon Balsamic Vinegar, caramelized

2 tablespoons Olive Oil

1 Leek, sliced thinly

A bunch of Kale (stems removed), chopped coarsely

8 medium Eggs, separated

2 tablespoons fresh Oregano, chopped

2 tablespoons fresh Basil, shredded

50 grams Butter

½ cup Parmesan Cheese, grated finely

6 slices Prosciutto, torn into pieces

Directions:

1. Preheat oven to 180° Celsius. Line tomatoes on a baking tray and drizzle with oil. Season with salt and pepper.

Roast tomatoes for 8 minutes or until tender. Drizzle with vinegar. Set aside covered to keep warm.

2. In a non-stick frying pan, heat the remaining oil and sauté the leeks. Stir until leeks are soft and almost brown. Add in kale leaves and stir until wilted. Season with salt and pepper. Put in a bowl and set aside.

3. In a mixing bowl, whisk the white eggs using an electric beater until soft peaks start to form. In a separate bowl, whisk egg yolks using a fork. Slowly fold egg yolk, basil and oregano into the beaten egg white.

4. Using the same pan you used for sautéing the leeks, melt butter over medium-low heat. Swirl to cover the entire bottom of the pan. Pour egg mixture and swirl until the base of the pan is covered with egg. Cook until the edges are set. Remove from heat and sprinkle kale and parmesan cheese on top. Bake for about 10 minutes or until golden brown. Top with prosciutto pieces. Serve with roasted tomatoes.

Chili Beef Con Red Beans

Ingredients:

1.4 kilos lean Beef, minced

2 cans (420 grams each) Red Kidney Beans, rinsed and drained

1/3 cup Vegetable Oil

4 medium Onions, chopped finely

4 cloves Garlic, chopped finely

2 Red Capsicums, deseeded, halved and cut into small pieces

2 teaspoons Chili Powder

2 teaspoons dried Oregano

2 teaspoons Cumin, ground

2 teaspoons Coriander, ground

1/3 cup Tomato Paste

800 grams fresh tomatoes, diced

Directions:

1. In a casserole, heat one teaspoon oil over medium heat. Mix in 1/3 of the minced beef and stir using wooden spoon. Mix until all lumps are broken apart and beef becomes brown. Transfer in a large bowl. Repeat the process until all the minced beef are sautéed in oil.

2. In the same casserole, heat the remaining oil and sauté the onions, garlic and capsicum. Add dried oregano, chili, coriander and cumin. Stir for 1 minute or until aroma starts to smell.

3. Pour in minced beef. Add tomato paste, tomato and kidney beans. Mix well and bring to a boil. Lower down heat to low. Cook for 20 minutes or until soup evaporates. Stir occasionally. Season with salt and pepper. Serve while hot.

Cheesy Gluten –Free Baked Macaroni

Ingredients:

16 ounces Gluten-Free Elbow Macaroni

A large bunch of Kale, stemmed, cut into ribbons

4 ounces White Cheddar, grated

4 ounces soft Goat Cheese, crumbled

Salt

Pepper

Directions:

1. Place some water in a large pot and add lots of salt (about 2 tablespoons or more). Bring to a boil and add elbow

macaroni. Stir for a minute to prevent the pieces from sticking together. Cook macaroni for 8 minutes.

2. While waiting for the pasta to cook, start setting up the sauce. In the bottom of a large, wide bowl, scatter goat cheese and white cheddar. Set aside.

3. Make sure the pasta is tender, but not too soft or al dente. Remove pasta from water and put on top of goat cheese and white cheddar. Save the water used for boiling the pasta.

4. Pour in about 1/3 to ½ cup of the boiled salted water in the bowl of macaroni. Place some kale on top. Set aside for 5 minutes. Mix the macaroni until everything is coated evenly with creamy sauce.

Note: You can substitute the goat cheese with cream cheese instead. For the cheddar, you can use Gruyere, Pecorino or any cheese of your choice. If you can't find Kale, you can use Spinach or Swiss Chard.

Sweet and Spicy Salad

Ingredients:

For the candied Pecans:

½ cup Pecans, raw

2 tablespoons Brown Sugar

2 tablespoons unsalted Butter

For the dressing:

2 teaspoons Maple Syrup

1 teaspoon Dijon Mustard

2 teaspoons Balsamic Vinegar

¼ cup extra-virgin Olive Oil

1 small Shallot, diced finely

Salt

Black Pepper, finely ground

1 Endive, leaves separated

2 hearts torn Frisee

1 Radicchio, leaves torn coarsely

1 sliced Red Pear

¼ cup Parmesan Cheese, shaved

Directions:

1. Heat a non-stick pan using medium heat. Stir in brown sugar and butter. Stir until melted and add pecans. Toss to coat the pecans evenly and cook for 1 minute. Turn off heat and place in a baking tray. Set aside.

2. In a large bowl, combine Dijon mustard, balsamic vinegar and shallots. Gently drizzle with olive oil while whisking to emulsify dressing mixture. Mix in maple syrup. Use salt and pepper as seasonings.

3. In a separate mixing bowl, toss the pear slices and greens together with the salad dressing. Sprinkle with Parmesan cheese and top with candied pecans.

Chapter 5 - Gluten-Free Diet For Weight Loss

If you need to lose weight and go gluten-free at the same time, these recipes are great for you.

Tomato Peach Salad

Ingredients:

3 medium Tomatoes, wedged

1 large Pear, deseeded and wedged

1 small Red Onion, sliced thinly

Brown Sugar

Salt

Pepper

Directions:

1. In a large mixing bowl, combine tomatoes and peach wedges.

2. Season with salt, pepper and brown sugar. Toss to coat ingredients evenly.

3. Top with thinly sliced onions. Serve and enjoy.

Simple Caesar Salad

Ingredients:

For the dressing:

2 cloves Garlic, minced

4 Anchovy fillets in oil

1 medium Lemon, juiced

1 tablespoon Worcestershire Sauce

Salt

Black Pepper, ground

1 Egg Yolk

¼ cup Olive Oil

1 large head Romaine Lettuce

Parmesan Cheese, shaved

Croutons

Directions:

1. In a blender, puree anchovies, minced garlic, Worcestershire sauce, lemon juice, egg yolk, salt and pepper.

2. Gently add olive oil into the mixture while blender is running. Blend until thick and shiny.

3. Wash lettuce and drain excess water. Tear the leaves using your hands and toss in a mixing bowl. Add the dressing and toss to cover the leaves evenly. Add in shaved parmesan cheese. Top with croutons.

Simple Mango-Jicama Salad

Ingredients:

1 large ripe Mango, peeled and cut into thin slices

1 medium Jicama, peeled and cut into long, thin strips

1 small red Onion, sliced thinly

1 small radish, cut into very thin slices

A bunch of Cilantro, chopped

1 teaspoon Cumin

Salt

Cayenne Pepper

1 tablespoon Olive Oil

2 tablespoons Lime Juice

Directions:

1. In a large mixing bowl, toss together the mango slices, Jicama strips, radish, onions and cilantro.

2. Add cumin and cayenne pepper. Drizzle with olive oil and lemon juice. Toss until ingredients are well-combined. Season with salt, toss and serve.

Yellow Salad

Ingredients:

½ cup Corn Kernels

1 medium Yellow squash, cut into thin, circular slices

6 pieces Yellow Grape Tomatoes, cut into halves

2 tablespoons Olive Oil

A bunch of fresh Basil leaves, chopped finely

Salt

Black Pepper, ground

Directions:

1. In a frying pan, heat olive oil over medium heat. Sauté corn kernels until tender. Mix in yellow squash slices and cook until soft.

2. Remove from heat and transfer in a large mixing bowl. Toss in yellow grape tomatoes. Season with salt and pepper. Toss once more to evenly season the ingredients. Sprinkle with chopped basil leaves. Serve.

Chapter 6 - Gluten-Free Diet For Blood Sugar Solutions

Diabetes and celiac disease are both autoimmune diseases. There are some cases wherein a person suffers from both diabetes and celiac disease. If you are suffering from both, then these recipes are perfect for you.

Breakfast Egg Muffins

Ingredients:

10 large eggs, separated

¾ cup reduced-fat Cheddar Cheese, shredded (you may use any cheese of your choice)

2 tablespoons plain Greek Yogurt

Salt

Black pepper, finely grounded

2 tablespoons Mushroom slices (canned)

1 onion Leek, chopped

1 small Green Bell Pepper, chopped

1 small Red Bell Pepper, chopped

2 medium Tomatoes, seeded and chopped

Directions:

1. Preheat your oven to 180° Celsius. Spray a 12-cup muffin tin with cooking spray. You may use individual muffin tins as long as you spray its inside to avoid sticking.

2. Place vegetables in each muffin tin. Leave enough space for the egg mixture.

3. In a mixing bowl, whisk egg whites with electric mixer until soft peaks form. In a separate bowl, whisk egg yolks until almost white in color and add Greek yogurt. Whisk until fluffy. Gently fold in egg yolk mixture into the whisked egg white.

4. Add egg mixture in the muffin tins filled with vegetables. Fill the muffin tins near the brim, but be careful not to put too much as the egg muffin will rise while cooking.

5. Bake for about 25 to 30 minutes or until the egg muffins have raised and brown on the sides.

6. Let cool and remove from tin. You may keep them in the refrigerator in a zip lock covered with paper towel to prevent sagging. Heat in microwave before serving.

Prosciutto-Wrapped Shrimps with Lemon Basil

Ingredients:

20 pieces large Shrimps, thawed and deveined

1 tablespoon fresh Basil, chopped

10 pieces Prosciutto, very thin slices

1 teaspoon extra virgin Olive Oil

½ teaspoon Lemon Zest

2 large Lemons, cut into 8 wedges

½ teaspoon Salt

1/8 teaspoon Black Pepper, finely ground

¼ teaspoon Red Pepper flakes

Cooking spray

Directions:

1. Preheat broiler. Combine basil, lemon zest, olive oil, red pepper flakes, black pepper and salt. Mix in shrimps and make sure each piece is well coated. Set aside.

2. Lay each Prosciutto slices on your work surface and cut into half, lengthwise. Wrap each shrimp pieces with the Prosciutto slices and leave the tail hanging out. Thread on skewers. Each skewer can thread 4 to 5 shrimps each.

3. Lightly coat broiling pan with cooking spray. Broil each side of the shrimp for 2 minutes. Lay hot on serving plate with lemon wedges.

Potato Soup

Ingredients:

1 tablespoon Olive Oil

1 medium Sweet Onion, diced

4 large Gold Potatoes, peeled and diced

2 cups Water

1 cup Coconut Milk

Salt

Ground Pepper

Nutmeg, ground

½ cup roasted Green Chili

Spring onions, chopped

Directions:

1. In a soup pot, heat olive oil over medium heat. Sauté onions until translucent. Add potatoes and pour 1 cup of water or enough to cover the potatoes.

2. Cover pot and boil over high heat until potatoes are soft. Add coconut milk and simmer for a few minutes. Remove from heat and cool.

3. Whip the soup with an immersion blender until smooth. Season with salt, pepper and a dash of nutmeg. Stir in roasted green chilies and return to heat. Simmer for a few minutes. Serve topped with spring onions.

Chapter 7 - Safe Gluten-Free Substitutes

Going on a gluten-free diet does not mean you have to skip the best things in life. There are safe substitutes for gluten-containing foods that are equally tasty, but more nutritious and safer to eat for people who suffer from celiac disease and gluten intolerance.

Here is the list of safe gluten-free substitutes:

- For bread crumbs – Substitute with corn meal for added crunch.

- For baking – Use Xanthan or Guar Gum when baking gluten-free goodies for them to rise and retain their shape.

- For flour – You can use rice flour, buckwheat flour, tapioca starch or sorghum instead. Millet flour, almond meal flour, coconut flour and potato flour are also great substitutes.

- For noodles – Use rice noodles or noodles made from beans.

- For pasta – You can use pasta made from rice, soy, corn, quinoa, or bean flour.

Fresh produce are mostly gluten-free except for grains such as rye, wheat, barley and triticale. Fruits and vegetables are the safest since they are all gluten-free.

If you are not suffering from celiac disease or gluten intolerance and you want to go gluten-free, watch out for products labeled as such. Since these products are already processed, some may contain more sugar or calories that are not good for your health.

Chapter 8 - Gluten-Free Slow Cooker Recipes

Slow cooker is best for soups, stews and casserole recipes. These are best enjoyed for lunch or dinner.

Slow Cooker Buttered Chicken

Ingredients:

4 Chicken thighs, skinned, deboned and cut into small pieces

40 grams Butter

3 cloves Garlic, minced

1 medium Onion, diced

1 tablespoon Curry Powder

1 tablespoon Indian Curry Paste

400ml Coconut Milk

140 grams Tomato Paste

1 teaspoon Garam Masala

2 Teaspoons Tandoori Masala

15 pods Green Cardamom

1 cup Yogurt, plain

2 tablespoons Vegetable Oil

Salt

Directions:

1. In a large frying pan, melt butter and add vegetable oil. Sauté onion, garlic and chicken until meat are all white.

2. Mix in curry powder, curry paste, tomato paste, garam masala and tandoori masala. Stir until tomato paste is smooth and no lumps appear.

3. Transfer into slow cooker and add yogurt, coconut milk and cardamom pods. Season with salt.

4. Cook on low for 6 to 8 hours or until chicken is soft and the sauce has reduced to a thicker consistency. Discard cardamom pods before serving.

Tip: To make it easier to discard the cardamom pods, insert needle with thread from end to end and make a ring-like shape. This way, you just need to fish out once and save time fishing out the pods one by one.

Slow Cooker Beef Stew

Ingredients:

2 lbs. grass-fed Beef, cubed

3 large Gold Potatoes, peeled and diced

3 large Carrots, peeled and diced

2 stalks Celery, chopped

5 cloves Garlic, chopped

1 cup Pearl Onions, trimmed and peeled

2 teaspoon dried Basil

1 Bay Leaf

Black Pepper, ground

4 cups Beef broth

1 tablespoon Balsamic Vinegar

1 cup Dry Red Table Wine

Directions:

1. Salt the beef cubes on all sides and set aside for a few minutes.

2. Set your slow cooker to high.

3. In a deep pot, heat olive oil over medium heat and brown the beef cubes on all sides. Transfer to the crock-pot.

4. Stir in pearl onions, garlic, carrots, potatoes and celery. Add wine and pour in broth.

5. Add all the herbs, balsamic vinegar and pepper. Stir and cover. Cook for 4 to 5 hours or until beef is soft and tender. Season with salt and pepper as needed. Serve while hot.

Chili Black Beans

3 cans (15 oz. each) Black Beans, washed and drained

1 can (15 oz.) refried Pinto Beans

1 lb lean Beef, ground

2 cups Tomatoes, deseeded and diced

1 quart Beef Stock

4 tablespoons Olive Oil

2 large Onions, chopped

2 tablespoons Chile Powder

2 tablespoons dried Cilantro

2 tablespoons Ancho Chili Powder

1 tablespoon Cumin, ground

¼ cup Lime Juice

1 medium Lime, diced

¾ cup fresh Cilantro, chopped

Low-fat Sour Cream (for serving)

Directions:

1. In a frying pan, heat 2 tablespoons olive oil and sauté onions until soft and almost brown. Transfer sautéed onions to the crock-pot.

2. In the same frying pan, sauté minced beef until brown. Add more olive oil if needed. Mix until lumps break up. Add sautéed beef in the crock-pot together with the onions. Cook in medium heat. Mix until well combined.

3. Meanwhile, in a saucepan, simmer beef stock until it is reduced to 2 cups. Whisk in refried beans so that it blends well into the stock. Add into the crock-pot.

4. While the stock is simmering, place the canned black beans in a colander and rinse on the sink until foam no longer appears. Add into the crock-pot together with refried beans, chili powder, diced tomatoes, dried cilantro, ancho chili powder and cumin powder.

5. Cook on low for 6 to 8 hours or until the beans are soft and all the flavors are well combined. Stir occasionally. When ready to serve, mix in lime juice and fresh cilantro. Simmer for 15 minutes. Serve hot with lime slices and top with chopped fresh cilantro and a dollop of low-fat sour cream.

Chapter 9 - Simple Gluten-Free Dessert Recipes

Going gluten-free also means having tasty, satisfying desserts that are healthy and delightful. Satisfy your sweet cravings with these simple, tasty desserts.

Apple Crisps

Ingredients:

6 Apples, peeled, cored and sliced

¾ cup Sorghum Flour (substitute with Brown Rice Flour)

2 teaspoons Tapioca Starch (substitute with Arrowroot Starch)

1 cup Quinoa Flakes

2 tablespoons Maple Syrup

1 cup Brown Sugar, organic

2 teaspoons Cinnamon, ground

1 teaspoon Ginger, ground

¾ cup Coconut Oil

½ teaspoon Salt

Butter (for greasing)

Directions:

1. Preheat oven to 180° Celsius. Grease an 8x11 baking dish with butter and set aside.

2. Place the sliced apples in a mixing bowl and sprinkle with lemon juice. Toss to coat evenly. Stir in maple syrup. Dust with tapioca starch and mix to coat the apple slices. Neatly arrange the coated apple slices into the greased baking dish.

3. In another mixing bowl, combine brown rice flour, quinoa flakes, brown sugar, ginger, cinnamon and salt. Whisk to blend well.

4. Add the coconut oil into the mixture in pieces. Use a whisker to cut the coconut oil into the flour mixture. Whisk until the mixture is even and sandy.

5. Spoon the mixture all over the top of the apple slices. Bake for 20 minutes. Loosely cover the baking dish with foil and bake for another 20 minutes or until apples are fork tender and the sides are starting to bubble.

6. Cool and serve.

Maple Cream Pumpkin Cupcakes

Ingredients:

1 cup Sorghum Flour (substitute with Brown Rice Flour)

¾ cup Potato Starch (substitute with Tapioca Starch)

¼ cup Almond Flour (substitute with Hazelnut Flour)

1 cup canned Pumpkin (organic)

1 cup Brown Sugar

½ cup Cane Sugar

1 teaspoon Baking Soda

1 teaspoon Baking Powder

1 teaspoon Xanthan Gum

1 teaspoon Cinnamon, ground

1 teaspoon Ginger, ground

½ teaspoon Salt

¼ teaspoon Nutmeg, ground

½ cup Coconut Oil

2 large Eggs, beaten

2 teaspoons Vanilla Extract

For the icing:

2 to 3 cups Powdered Sugar

¼ cup Cream Cheese

2 to 4 tablespoons Maple Syrup

Directions:

1. Preheat oven to 180° Celsius. Line a 12-cup muffin tin with cupcake liners.

2. Mix together all dry ingredients in a large mixing bowl.

3. Use whisker to cut coconut oil into pieces and slowly add into the bowl of dry ingredients. Continue whisking until mixture becomes sandy.

4. Add eggs, vanilla and pumpkin. Beat using electric mixer set to medium high for 1 to 2 minutes or until batter is stretchy and smooth.

5. Spoon the batter into each cupcake liners. Smooth the top of each cupcake.

6. Bake for 25 minutes or until cupcake tops are firm. Cool until warm enough for you to handle. Remove from baking pan and transfer on a wire rack to cool for an hour.

7. While cooling the cupcakes, start making your icing. In a mixing bowl, beat together cream cheese and powdered sugar. Beat in maple syrup, adding a tablespoon at a time until frosting is smooth and soft.

8. Beat for another 1 to 2 minutes on medium-high or until frosting is fluffy, glossy and smooth. Cover and chill in the refrigerator while waiting for the cupcakes to be cool enough for frosting.

9. Frost each cupcake using an icing knife or decorate it as you wish. Chill to allow the frosting to set. Serve.

Chapter 10 - Paleo Diet &Paleo Smoothies For Gluten-Free Living

Paleo diet and gluten-free diet can be incorporated due to their great similarities. Below are Paleo-approved recipes that are also gluten-free.

Chicken Vegetable Stir-Fry

Ingredients:

1 lb free-range Chicken breasts, skinned and deboned

2 medium heads Broccoli, sliced

2 medium Carrots, sliced

2 heads Baby Bok Choy, sliced into 1-inch crosswise strips

1 small Zucchini, sliced

4 ounces Shiitake Mushrooms, stemmed and sliced thinly

1 medium Onion, chopped finely

2 tablespoons Coconut Oil

2 tablespoon toasted Sesame Oil

1 ½ cups Water

1 tablespoon Honey

2 tablespoons Ume Plum Vinegar

2 tablespoons Arrowroot Powder

Directions:

1. Rinse chicken breasts and pat dry with paper towel. Slice into 1-inch cubes. Place on a plate and set aside.

2. In a large skillet, heat coconut oil over medium heat. Sauté onion until translucent. Stir in chicken, carrots and broccoli. Cook until tender.

3. Add mushrooms, bokchoy and zucchini. Season with salt and sauté for five minutes. Pour 1 cup water and cover the skillet. Cook until vegetables are wilted.

4. In a small bowl, dissolve arrowroot powder using the remaining ½ cup of water. Add the mixture to the vegetables and stir until sauce becomes thick and glossy. Mix in vinegar, sesame oil and honey. Serve while hot.

Beef-Wrapped Asparagus

Ingredients:

1lb lean grass-fed Beef

25 to 30 stalks Asparagus, ends trimmed

1 clove Garlic, minced

½ teaspoon Ginger, peeled and grated

½ teaspoon dried Red Pepper flakes

½ teaspoon Sesame Seeds

½ teaspoon Sea salt

½ teaspoon Pepper, ground

1 tablespoon Sesame Oil

1 teaspoon Honey

1 tablespoon Pineapple Juice, unsweetened

1 teaspoon Fish Sauce

1 teaspoon extra-virgin Olive Oil

½ cup Coconut Aminos

Directions:

1. Freeze the beef for 45 minutes to allow easier slicing of the meat.

2. While waiting, prepare the marinade. In a mixing bowl, combine garlic, ginger and red pepper flakes. Stir in coconut aminos, honey, sesame oil, fish sauce and pineapple juice. Mix thoroughly and set aside.

3. Put the beef meat out from freezer. Cut into very thin strips. Pour marinade over the beef strips and marinade for 6 to 8 hours in the refrigerator.

4. Preheat grill to medium heat. Meanwhile, prepare your asparagus. Rub olive oil all over the asparagus stalks and individually wrap with marinated beef strips.

5. Season with salt and pepper and sprinkle with sesame seeds.

6. Grill over medium heat for 6 minutes. Turn occasionally to ensure even cooking.

Sweet Green Smoothie

Ingredients:

¾ cup unsweetened, plain Almond Milk

1 tablespoon Flaxseed, ground

A pinch of Sea Salt

1 packet Stevia

1 teaspoon fresh Ginger, grated

45 grams organic Baby Spinach

1 Persian Cucumber (reserve 3 thin slices), ends trimmed and cut into chunks

1 medium Pear, cored and quartered (freeze before using)

Directions:

1. In a blender, combine almond milk, flaxseed, stevia, ginger, spinach, cucumber and pear. Season with salt. Blend until smooth.

2. Pour in a serving glass topped with the cucumber slices. Serve right away.

Almond Coco Banana Smoothie

Ingredients:

½ cup unsweetened, plain Almond Milk

2 tablespoons Coconut Milk

¾ teaspoon Coconut Extract

1/8 teaspoon Almond Extract

1 tablespoon unsweetened Cocoa Powder

½ Banana, peeled, chopped and frozen

1 Medjool Dates, pitted and chopped

A pinch of Sea Salt

1 packet Stevia

2 tablespoons unsweetened Coconut, shredded (as garnish)

Ice Cubes

Directions:

1. Place all ingredients in a blender except for the shredded coconut and ice cubes. Blend until smooth.

2. Add ice cubes and pulse until broken down into pieces.

3. Pour in serving glass and mix shredded coconut. Sprinkle with leftover shredded coconut on top. Serve right away.

Conclusion

Thank you again for purchasing this book on eating a Gluten-Free Diet!

I am extremely excited to pass this information along to you, and I am so happy that you now have read and can hopefully implement these strategies going forward.

I hope this book was able to help you understand what a Gluten-Free Diet is and how to eat healthy and live healthy, Gluten-Free, within budget.

The next step is to get started using this information and to hopefully live disease-free and better life!

Please don't be someone who just reads this information and doesn't apply it, the strategies in this book will only benefit you if you use them!

If you know of anyone else that could benefit from the information presented here please inform them of this book.

Finally, if you enjoyed this book and feel it has added value to your life in any way, please take the time to share your thoughts and post a review on Amazon. It'd be greatly appreciated!

Thank you and good luck!

Preview Of:

Ultimate Alkaline Foods Guide!

<u>Alkaline Foods</u>

Learn How To Alkalize Your Body With This PH Balance Diet And Superfoods Guide To Increase Your Energy, Fat Loss, Natural Beauty And Health!

Introduction

I want to thank you and congratulate you for purchasing the book, *Alkaline Foods: Ultimate Alkaline Foods Guide! Learn How To Alkalize Your Body With This PH Balance Diet and Superfoods Guide to Increase Your Energy, Fat Loss, Natural Beauty and Health!*

This book contains proven steps and strategies on how you can change your diet to something healthier and better for you in the long-term. With the alkaline diet, your body will function better. The diet plan can also help raise your energy level and improve your immunity to different illnesses as well as infections.

You may not notice it but the foods that you consume on a daily basis have a direct effect on your body, starting with how energetic you are to how your skin looks. The thing is that the average Western diet is actually highly acidic and this causes a number of different health problems for people with heart diseases and obesity being the most common. However, with a simple diet change you can avoid these completely.

We hope that this book can provide you with all the information that you need when it comes to getting started with the alkaline diet and use it to enjoy a healthier and more satisfying life.

Thanks again for purchasing this book, I hope you enjoy it!

Chapter 1: What Are Acidic Foods And How Do They Affect Your Body?

When it comes to maintaining your overall health and well-being, the foods that you consume regularly play a significant role. Too much of acidic foods can bring about a number of health issues just as too much alkalinity can bring about an imbalance. Making sure that your body's blood pH stays within the right level is imperative if you want to stay healthy and avoid different health complications. To do that, however, you will need an understanding of what alkaline and acidic foods are along with the effects they have on your body.

What are Acidic Foods and How Do they Affect your Body?

Contrary to what most people think, simply eating acidic foods will not immediately cause your blood, stomach or body to become acidic too. It is the process of digestion that eventually takes it up a notch and causes damage on your body slowly but surely. During digestion, the stomach secretes hydrochloric acid (a highly acidic substance) and this, mixed with the acid in the foods you eat, will make you feel ill.

Here's a quick summary of some of the most common problems that are associated to having a highly acidic diet:

- If left untreated, high amounts of acid in your body will also begin to move into your tissues and joints. This will not only cause damage but some discomfort as well. In more advanced cases, joint pain is not an unusual symptom. Your bones will also start to weaken more and you will become more prone to bone-related issues such as osteopenia.

- Acidity can also bring about number of skin-related issues; eczema is the most common skin disorder of all. Too much acidity can also lead to brittle hair, dry skin, as well as a number of oral issues. Bleeding gums and bad breath are also common symptoms of a highly acidic diet.

- There are also certain heart issues that may arise from having a highly acidic diet. Two of the most common symptoms would be an increase in your heart rate and arrhythmia. Of course, a highly acidic diet that is coupled with a lack of proper exercise can certainly lead to even greater issues.

- When it comes to the negative effects of too much acidity to your body, your intestinal and gastric systems will take the hardest hit. In some cases, vomiting, nausea, diarrhea, heartburn and acid reflux may be experienced. This is especially so if there's a major imbalance in your blood PH. None of these are a walk in the park and they usually happen out of the blue as well.

Thanks For Previewing My Exciting Book Entitled:

"Alkaline Foods: Ultimate Alkaline Foods Guide! Learn How To Alkalize Your Body With This PH Balance Diet And Superfoods Guide To Increase Your Energy, Fat Loss, Natural Beauty And Health!"

To purchase this book, simply go to the Amazon Kindle store and simply search:

"ALKALINE FOODS"

Then just scroll down until you see my book. You will know it is mine because you will see my name "Sarah Brooks" underneath the title.

Alternatively, you can visit my author page on Amazon to see this book and other work I have done. Thanks so much, and please don't forget your free bonuses

DON'T LEAVE YET! - CHECK OUT YOUR FREE BONUSES BELOW!

Free Bonus Offer: Get Free Access To The www.LiveFitVIP.com VIP Newsletter!

Once you enter your email address you will immediately get free access to this awesome newsletter!

But wait, right now if you join now for free you will also get free access to the "The 7 Keys To Body Transformation" free EBook!

To claim both your FREE VIP NEWSLETTER MEMBERSHIP and your FREE BONUS EBook on THE 7 KEYS TO BODY TRANSFORMATION!

Just Go To:

www.liveFitVIP.com

www.ingramcontent.com/pod-product-compliance
Lightning Source LLC
Chambersburg PA
CBHW070844290526
45795CB00002B/972